Plant- Based cooking made easy

Delicious recipe for a healthier you

By

Sylvia ken

TABLE OF CONTENTS

INTRODUCTION

In a world where culinary choices seem limitless, the rise of plant-based cooking has captured the attention and palates of people from all walks of life. The allure of vibrant vegetables, legumes, fruits, nuts, and whole grains has sparked a revolution in the kitchen. Whether you're a seasoned chef or a novice home cook, embarking on a journey into plant-based cooking offers a multitude of benefits.

The world of cooking is a vast and ever-evolving realm, offering endless possibilities and flavors to explore. Amid this culinary landscape, plant-based cooking has emerged as a vibrant and rewarding path, captivating the hearts and taste buds of those who dare to venture into its rich terrain.

The journey into plant-based cooking isn't just about changing what's on your plate; it's about transforming the way you think about food, health, and the environment. It's a journey that brings with it a host of benefits, not only for you but for the planet we all call home.

The Benefits of Plant-Based Cooking

The opening chapter of this book delves into the myriad advantages of plant-based cooking. Beyond the flavors and textures that tantalize the taste buds, the benefits extend to our health, the environment, and even our wallets. Discover how adopting a plant-based lifestyle can lead to improved well-being, reduced environmental impact, and cost-effective meal planning.

Plant-based cooking is more than just a dietary choice; it's a lifestyle that offers a multitude of advantages. We'll explore how embracing plant-based ingredients can lead to improved health. Discover the science behind lower cholesterol levels, reduced risk of chronic diseases, and increased vitality as you explore the world of whole foods.

Beyond the individual health benefits, plant-based cooking extends its positive impact to the world around us. You'll learn how adopting this approach can significantly reduce your carbon footprint, conserve natural resources, and contribute to a more sustainable future. It's a way of eating that aligns with the values of environmental responsibility and compassion for all living beings.

Getting Started with Plant-Based Ingredients

Transitioning to plant-based cooking can seem daunting if you're not familiar with the ingredients that form the foundation of this culinary style. Fear not! This chapter will guide you through the essentials of plant-based ingredients. From selecting fresh produce to exploring protein-rich alternatives like tofu and tempeh, helping you decipher the labels, pick the freshest produce, and explore the delightful world of grains, legumes, and plant-based proteins.you'll gain the knowledge and confidence to navigate the aisles of your local grocery store with ease.

By the time you've completed this section, you'll not only understand the nutritional value of each ingredient but also feel confident navigating your local grocery store or farmers' market. With your newfound knowledge, you'll be ready to embark on culinary adventures that are both delicious and nutritious.

Essential Kitchen Tools and Equipment

Equipping your kitchen with the right tools and appliances is key to making plant-based cooking a breeze. We'll walk you through a list of must-have kitchen items that will simplify your cooking process. From blenders that create velvety smooth sauces to versatile cookware that can handle a variety of dishes, we'll provide you with a comprehensive list of essentials. You'll soon see how these tools can streamline your cooking process, making plant-based meals not only easy but also enjoyable to prepare.

As we embark on this plant-based culinary journey together, remember that you're not just changing what you eat; you're embracing a lifestyle that has far-reaching benefits. So, let's dive into the vibrant world of plant-based cooking, starting with an exploration of its myriad advantages, an introduction to essential ingredients, and the tools that will empower you to create flavorful, satisfying, and nourishing dishes.

CHAPTER 1: Breakfast Delights

Breakfast is often hailed as the most important meal of the day, and when it comes to plant-based options, it's a time to savor a wide array of flavors and textures. In this chapter, we'll explore breakfast delights that not only jumpstart your day with energy but also tantalize your taste buds, making every morning something to look forward to.

As you dive into the world of breakfast delights in this chapter, you'll discover that plant-based cooking doesn't compromise on flavor or satisfaction. In fact, it opens up a world of possibilities where health and indulgence go hand in hand. So, get ready to awaken your senses and start your day with a smile as you explore the recipes for scrumptious smoothie bowls, hearty vegan pancakes, and the convenience of overnight oats with fruits and nuts.

Scrumptious Smoothie Bowls

Let's begin with the art of creating the perfect smoothie bowl. These visually stunning creations are a symphony of colors and flavors. Learn how to blend creamy plant-based yogurt, ripe fruits, and nutrient-packed greens into a thick, spoonable delight. We'll guide you through the process of assembling your masterpiece, adding toppings like fresh berries, crunchy granola, and a drizzle of honey or maple syrup for that extra touch of sweetness. With smoothie bowls, you'll experience breakfast as a celebration of health and taste, all in one delicious package.

Smoothie bowls are the epitome of breakfast creativity. Not only do they offer a refreshing and nutritious start to your day, but they also provide an artistic canvas for culinary expression.

The Art of Blending

Creating the perfect smoothie bowl begins with mastering the art of blending. Start with a base of plant-based yogurt or milk – almond, soy, or coconut, for instance – to achieve that creamy texture. Add a generous handful of fresh or frozen fruits, such as bananas, berries, or mango, for a burst of flavor and natural sweetness. Don't forget to toss in a handful of leafy greens like spinach or kale to sneak in some extra nutrients without altering the taste.

Balancing Flavors and Textures

The magic of smoothie bowls lies in the balance of flavors and textures. To enhance the sweetness, you can drizzle in a touch of honey, maple syrup, or agave nectar. For a little zing, a squeeze of citrus juice or a sprinkle of zest can work wonders. To elevate the creaminess, consider adding a spoonful of nut butter or avocado. Blend until smooth, and don't hesitate to taste along the way, adjusting the ingredients to suit your palate.

Toppings Galore

What truly sets smoothie bowls apart is the medley of toppings that adorn them. This is where you can let your creativity shine. From fresh berries, sliced bananas, and kiwi to a sprinkling of chia seeds, shredded coconut, or chopped nuts, the choices are endless. These toppings add not only visual appeal but also a delightful mix of flavors and textures that make each spoonful a new adventure.

Presentation Matters

In the world of smoothie bowls, presentation is key. Pour your blended mixture into a bowl and use the back of a spoon to create decorative swirls or patterns on the surface. Then, arrange your chosen toppings with care, ensuring an even distribution of colors and textures. The result is a visually stunning work of art that's almost too beautiful to eat – almost.

A Wholesome Breakfast

Beyond their artistic appeal, smoothie bowls offer a wholesome breakfast that's rich in vitamins, minerals, and fiber. They provide a satisfying combination of carbohydrates, healthy fats, and plant-based proteins to fuel your morning. Whether you're looking to boost your energy, improve digestion, or simply enjoy a delightful breakfast, smoothie bowls check all the boxes.

As you explore the world of scrumptious smoothie bowls, you'll quickly realize that they're not just a breakfast option – they're a delightful way to express your culinary flair while nourishing your body. So, grab your blender, unleash your creativity, and start your day with a bowl of vibrant, nutrient-packed goodness.

Hearty Vegan Pancakes

Who can resist the aroma of freshly cooked pancakes wafting through the kitchen on a lazy weekend morning? The good news is that you don't have to give up this beloved

breakfast tradition when you embrace
plant-based cooking. We'll reveal the secrets
to creating fluffy and satisfying vegan
pancakes. These pancakes are not only
delicious but also wholesome, often featuring
whole grain flours, mashed bananas, or
applesauce as key ingredients. Stack them
high, drizzle with your favorite syrup or fruit
compote, and enjoy a guilt-free indulgence
that leaves you nourished and ready to tackle
the day.

Plant-Based Substitutions

Traditional pancake recipes typically call for
eggs and dairy milk. In vegan pancakes, these
ingredients are replaced with plant-based
alternatives. Instead of eggs, you can use
ingredients like mashed bananas, applesauce,
flaxseed meal, or silken tofu to bind the
batter and add moisture. Opt for almond

milk, soy milk, or oat milk to replace dairy milk, and you'll achieve the same creamy consistency that makes pancakes so irresistible.

The Perfect Pancake Batter

Creating the perfect vegan pancake batter is all about achieving the right balance of wet and dry ingredients. Start with a blend of all-purpose flour and whole wheat flour for a heartier, more nutritious pancake. Add a touch of sweetness with a drizzle of maple syrup or a pinch of sugar. A dash of vanilla extract and a hint of cinnamon can elevate the flavor profile.

Cooking to Perfection

The key to fluffy vegan pancakes is to avoid overmixing the batter. Stir it just until the dry ingredients are incorporated; a few lumps are perfectly fine. Preheat your non-stick skillet or griddle over medium-low heat, and lightly grease it with coconut oil or a vegan cooking spray. Ladle the batter onto the hot surface and allow it to spread naturally. When bubbles form on the surface and the edges start to set, it's time to flip the pancakes. Cook until both sides are golden brown and the centers are cooked through.

Endless Variations

Vegan pancakes are incredibly versatile, and you can get creative with your add-ins. Toss in fresh blueberries, diced apples, chocolate chips, or chopped nuts for added flavor and texture. You can also experiment with different flours, such as spelt or buckwheat, to create unique pancake variations to suit your taste.

Healthy Indulgence

One of the beautiful aspects of vegan pancakes is that they can be both indulgent and nutritious. Whole grains, fruit additions, and natural sweeteners make them a wholesome breakfast option. Pair them with a dollop of dairy-free yogurt, a drizzle of pure maple syrup, or a handful of fresh berries for a breakfast that satisfies your cravings while nourishing your body.

As you dive into the world of hearty vegan pancakes, you'll discover that making this breakfast classic plant-based doesn't mean sacrificing flavor or comfort. In fact, it opens up a world of delicious possibilities, where you can enjoy a stack of pancakes guilt-free and embrace a cruelty-free breakfast that's as hearty as it is satisfying. So, preheat that skillet, mix up some batter, and get ready to savor the joy of homemade vegan pancakes.

Overnight Oats with Fruits and Nuts

For those mornings when time is of the essence, overnight oats are a lifesaver. Prepare them the night before, and wake up to a nutritious and filling breakfast that requires no cooking. In this section, we'll show you how to combine rolled oats with plant-based milk, a variety of toppings such as fresh fruits, nuts, and seeds, and a touch of sweetness from natural sources like maple syrup or agave nectar. Overnight oats are not only convenient but also highly customizable, allowing you to create a breakfast that suits your taste and nutritional preferences.

This no-cook, make-ahead meal not only simplifies your morning routine but also delivers a wholesome and delightful start to your day. In this section, we'll delve into the art of preparing overnight oats with fruits and nuts, unlocking the secrets to this convenient and nutritious breakfast option.

The Beauty of Preparation

The magic of overnight oats lies in the preparation. Before you go to bed, take just a few minutes to assemble your ingredients in a jar or container. Begin with rolled oats as the base – they're hearty and create a satisfying texture when soaked overnight. Add your choice of plant-based milk, such as almond, soy, or coconut, in a ratio that suits your desired consistency. A touch of sweetness from natural sources like maple syrup or agave nectar complements the oats perfectly.

The Art of Customization

What sets overnight oats apart is their versatility. You can customize them to suit your taste and nutritional preferences. Feel free to toss in a handful of fresh or dried fruits like sliced bananas, diced apples, or raisins. Add a variety of nuts and seeds for crunch and healthy fats – options range from chopped almonds and walnuts to chia seeds and flaxseed. A dash of cinnamon or a drop of vanilla extract can infuse your oats with even more flavor.

The Overnight Magic

As you mix your ingredients together and seal the container, a subtle transformation begins overnight. The oats absorb the liquid, softening into a delightful, pudding-like texture. The fruits release their natural sweetness, and the nuts and seeds provide a satisfying crunch. When you open the container in the morning, you're greeted with a ready-to-eat breakfast that's both convenient and nutritious.

The Grab-and-Go Breakfast

Perhaps the most significant advantage of overnight oats is their grab-and-go nature. As you rush through your morning routine, simply grab your pre-prepared jar of oats from the fridge, give it a quick stir, and enjoy a nourishing breakfast at your desk, on the commute, or wherever your day takes you. No cooking, no fuss – just pure breakfast bliss.

Health and Satisfaction in a Jar

Beyond their convenience, overnight oats are a nutritional powerhouse. They provide a hearty dose of fiber, which helps keep you full and satisfied throughout the morning. The combination of fruits, nuts, and seeds offers a variety of essential vitamins, minerals, and healthy fats. Plus, they're a fantastic source of energy to fuel your day.

As you embrace the world of overnight oats with fruits and nuts, you'll discover that this breakfast option is not just about simplicity; it's about creating a delicious and nutritious morning ritual that supports your busy lifestyle. So, start preparing your own customized jars of overnight oats, and wake up to a wholesome and satisfying breakfast that sets the tone for a successful day ahead.

CHAPTER 2: Appetizing Appetizers

Appetizers are the opening act of any memorable meal, setting the stage for what's to come. In this section, we'll explore a trio of appetizers that are not only delicious but also perfect for gatherings, parties, or simply elevating your everyday dining experience.

Appetizers, often referred to as the "teasers" of the culinary world, hold a special place in the hearts of food enthusiasts and home cooks alike. They mark the beginning of a culinary journey, igniting anticipation and delight with every bite. In this section, we'll dive deeper into the world of appetizing appetizers, exploring a trio of delectable options that will not only whet your appetite but also awaken your palate to a symphony of flavors and textures.

Before the main course takes center stage, appetizers play a crucial role in preparing your taste buds for the culinary adventure ahead. They offer a tantalizing glimpse of what's to come, warming up your senses and building excitement for the meal that follows. Whether you're hosting a gathering of friends and family or simply seeking to elevate your everyday dining experience, these appetizers are the perfect opening act.

Within this section, we'll unveil a trio of appetizers that showcase both creativity and flavor. Guacamole and salsa are a dynamic duo that effortlessly combines the creamy richness of avocados with the zesty freshness of tomatoes and herbs. Stuffed mushrooms offer an elegant option, showcasing the versatility of this humble fungi with a range of delectable fillings. Finally, crispy baked sweet potato fries bring a satisfying crunch and a hint of natural sweetness to your appetizer repertoire.

One of the remarkable qualities of appetizers is their versatility. These dishes are easily customizable to suit your taste preferences and dietary choices. Whether you're a fan of bold, spicy flavors or prefer something milder and comforting, these appetizers provide a canvas for your culinary creativity. You can adapt them to accommodate vegan, vegetarian, or omnivorous diets, ensuring that everyone at your table can indulge in the joy of appetizing appetizers.

As you explore the recipes and techniques in this section, you'll discover that appetizers aren't just about tickling your taste buds — they're a culinary prelude that sets the stage for a memorable dining experience. These dishes are perfect for sharing, sparking conversation, and creating a sense of togetherness. Whether you're celebrating a special occasion or simply savoring the everyday moments, these appetizers will elevate your meals to a whole new level of enjoyment.

So, let the curtain rise on a world of appetizing appetizers, where the flavors are bold, the textures are enticing, and the culinary possibilities are endless. Get ready to tantalize your taste buds with guacamole and salsa, stuffed mushrooms, and crispy baked sweet potato fries.

Guacamole and Salsa

Few appetizers can rival the classic combination of guacamole and salsa. Guacamole, with its creamy avocado base, is a luxurious dip that's both rich in flavor and healthy fats. To prepare it, simply mash ripe avocados and blend them with diced tomatoes, onions, cilantro, lime juice, and a dash of salt and pepper. The result is a vibrant green dip that's both refreshing and satisfying.

Salsa, on the other hand, offers a burst of freshness and zing. Made from ripe tomatoes, onions, jalapeños, cilantro, and lime juice, it provides a delightful contrast to the creamy guacamole. Whether you prefer it mild or with an extra kick, salsa adds a layer of excitement to your appetizer platter.

Guacamole Recipe

Ingredients:

- 3 ripe avocados

- 1 medium tomato, diced
- 1/2 cup finely chopped red onion
- 1/4 cup fresh cilantro, chopped
- 1-2 cloves garlic, minced
- 1 lime, juiced
- Salt and pepper to taste

Instructions:

1. **Prepare the Avocados:** Cut the avocados in half, remove the seeds, and scoop the flesh into a mixing bowl.

2. **Mash the Avocado:** Use a fork or a potato masher to mash the avocado to your preferred level of smoothness. Some like it chunky, while others prefer it smoother.

3. **Add the Lime Juice:** Squeeze the juice of one lime over the mashed avocado. Lime not only adds flavor but also helps prevent the guacamole from browning.

4. **Add the Garlic:** Mince the garlic cloves and add them to the bowl. Adjust the amount of garlic to your taste preference; one to two cloves usually work well.

5. **Mix in the Tomato and Onion:** Add the diced tomato and finely chopped red onion to the bowl. These ingredients provide texture and a fresh, crisp taste to the guacamole.

6. **Incorporate the Cilantro:** Chop the fresh cilantro finely and add it to the mixture. Cilantro adds a delightful herbal note to the guacamole.

7. **Season to Taste:** Sprinkle in salt and pepper, then gently fold all the ingredients together. Start with a small amount of salt and adjust to your liking.

8. **Taste and Adjust:** Take a taste test. If you prefer more acidity, you can add additional lime juice. If it needs more seasoning, add a pinch of salt or a dash of pepper.

9. **Serve:** Transfer the guacamole to a serving bowl. You can garnish it with a few extra cilantro leaves or a slice of lime for presentation.

10. **Enjoy:** Serve your homemade guacamole with tortilla chips, tacos, burritos, or as a condiment for various dishes. It's best enjoyed fresh, but you can cover it with plastic wrap, ensuring the wrap touches the surface of the guacamole to minimize browning, and store it in the refrigerator for a short period.

Salsa Recipe

Ingredients:

- 4-5 ripe tomatoes, diced
- 1/2 cup red onion, finely chopped
- 1/4 cup fresh cilantro, chopped
- 1-2 jalapeño or serrano peppers, finely
chopped (adjust for desired spiciness)
- 2 cloves garlic, minced
- Juice of 1 lime
- Salt and pepper to taste

Instructions:

1. **Prepare the Tomatoes:** Dice the ripe
tomatoes and place them in a mixing bowl.

2. **Add the Onion:** Finely chop the red onion
and add it to the tomatoes.

3. **Incorporate the Cilantro:** Chop the fresh cilantro finely and mix it into the bowl with the tomatoes and onion.

4. **Add the Peppers:** For a mild salsa, remove the seeds and membranes from the jalapeño or serrano peppers, then finely chop them. For a spicier version, leave some or all of the seeds and membranes intact. Add the chopped peppers to the bowl.

5. **Garlic and Lime Juice:** Mince the garlic cloves and add them to the mixture. Squeeze the juice of one lime over the ingredients.

6. **Season and Mix:** Sprinkle salt and pepper over the mixture, then gently fold all the ingredients together.

7. **Taste and Adjust:** Taste the salsa and adjust the seasoning if needed. You can add

more lime juice, salt, or pepper according to your taste.

8. **Chill (Optional):** If time allows, refrigerate the salsa for 30 minutes to an hour before serving to allow the flavors to meld.

9. **Serve:** Transfer the salsa to a serving bowl, and it's ready to be enjoyed.

10. **Enjoy:** Serve your homemade salsa with tortilla chips, tacos, grilled meats, or as a vibrant condiment. It's a fresh and flavorful addition to any meal.

These guacamole and salsa recipes are versatile, allowing you to customize them to suit your preferred level of spiciness and taste. They're perfect for sharing at gatherings, dipping with tortilla chips, or enhancing a variety of dishes. Enjoy the vibrant flavors of Mexico with these homemade delights!

Together, guacamole and salsa create a culinary synergy that's hard to resist. The creamy richness of guacamole balances the zesty punch of salsa, resulting in a perfect pairing. When served side by side, they provide a spectrum of flavors and textures that cater to a wide range of preferences. Each dip complements the other, inviting you to create your own unique combination with every bite.

Guacamole and salsa aren't just appetizers; they're symbols of culinary tradition and celebration. They bring people together, whether at festive gatherings, casual picnics, or intimate dinners. Their bright colors, bold flavors, and fresh ingredients evoke the spirit of joy and togetherness, making them the perfect choice for any occasion.

Stuffed Mushrooms

Stuffed mushrooms are a savory delight that combines earthy mushroom caps with a variety of flavorful fillings. Start by removing the stems from large mushroom caps and brushing them with a bit of olive oil. Then, choose your filling – it could be a mixture of breadcrumbs, garlic, herbs, and vegan cheese for a comforting option, or a blend of spinach, tofu, and sundried tomatoes for a more complex flavor profile. Stuff the caps generously and bake until they're tender and golden. These bite-sized morsels make for an impressive appetizer that's sure to disappear quickly.

Stuffed mushrooms are a culinary gem, an appetizer that marries the earthy flavors of mushrooms with a medley of flavorful fillings. These bite-sized delights have been a favorite at gatherings and events for generations, offering a delightful combination of umami richness and creative possibilities. In this section, we'll explore the art of preparing stuffed mushrooms, including a detailed recipe to help you master this classic appetizer.

The Perfect Mushroom

Before diving into the recipe, it's essential to select the right mushrooms. Cremini or white button mushrooms are popular choices due to their size and flavor. Look for firm, fresh mushrooms with smooth caps and intact stems. Avoid mushrooms that are overly mature or have signs of bruising.

Stuffed Mushrooms Recipe

Ingredients:

- 20-24 medium-sized cremini or white button mushrooms
- 1/4 cup olive oil
- 1/2 cup finely chopped onion
- 2 cloves garlic, minced
- 1/2 cup breadcrumbs (regular or gluten-free)
- 1/4 cup grated vegan Parmesan cheese (optional)
- 2 tablespoons fresh parsley, chopped
- Salt and pepper to taste

Instructions:

1. **Prepare the Mushrooms:** Carefully remove the stems from the mushrooms by gently twisting them. Set aside the caps, and finely chop the stems.

2. **Preheat the Oven:** Preheat your oven to 375°F (190°C). While the oven is heating, line a baking sheet with parchment paper.

3. **Prepare the Filling:** In a skillet, heat the olive oil over medium heat. Add the chopped mushroom stems and onions. Sauté until the onions are translucent and the mushroom stems have released their moisture, about 5-7 minutes. Stir in the minced garlic and cook for an additional minute.

4. **Create the Filling:** Remove the skillet from the heat. Stir in the breadcrumbs, grated vegan Parmesan cheese (if using), and fresh parsley. Season the mixture with salt and pepper to taste. The mixture should have a slightly moist consistency that holds together.

5. **Fill the Mushroom Caps:** Using a spoon, generously fill each mushroom cap with the

prepared filling. Press the filling gently to pack it into the caps.

6. **Bake the Stuffed Mushrooms:** Arrange the stuffed mushrooms on the prepared baking sheet. Place them in the preheated oven and bake for approximately 20-25 minutes or until the mushrooms are tender and the filling is golden brown.

7. **Serve:** Once baked, remove the stuffed mushrooms from the oven and let them cool slightly. Arrange them on a serving platter, garnish with additional fresh parsley if desired, and serve hot.

Variations and Tips:

- Feel free to experiment with the filling by adding ingredients like chopped spinach, sun-dried tomatoes, or diced bell peppers.

- If you prefer a dairy-free version, skip the vegan Parmesan cheese, or substitute it with nutritional yeast for a cheesy flavor.
- Stuffed mushrooms are an excellent make-ahead appetizer. You can prepare them up to a day in advance, refrigerate them, and then bake them just before serving.
- To serve as an hors d'oeuvre, consider pairing stuffed mushrooms with a dipping sauce, such as a garlic aioli or a balsamic reduction.

Stuffed mushrooms are a versatile appetizer that's sure to impress your guests or add elegance to any meal. They offer endless possibilities for customization, making them a beloved choice for both novice and experienced home cooks. Enjoy the delightful flavors and textures of this classic dish!

Crispy Baked Sweet Potato Fries

For those who crave a little crunch with their appetizers, crispy baked sweet potato fries are the perfect choice. These fries offer a healthier alternative to traditional potato fries and are incredibly simple to prepare. The natural sweetness of sweet potatoes, combined with the savory seasonings, creates a winning flavor combination that's hard to resist.

Crispy baked sweet potato fries are the perfect combination of sweet, savory, and crunchy. These fries are not only a healthier alternative to traditional deep-fried potatoes but also a delightful side dish or snack that's easy to make at home. In this section, we'll explore the art of preparing crispy baked sweet potato fries, complete with a detailed recipe that will help you achieve that perfect balance of tenderness and crunch.

Choosing the Right Sweet Potatoes

Selecting the right sweet potatoes is crucial to achieving the desired texture and flavor. Look for sweet potatoes that are firm and have smooth, unblemished skins. The orange-fleshed variety, often labeled as "yams," is commonly used for sweet potato fries due to their natural sweetness and vibrant color.

Crispy Baked Sweet Potato Fries Recipe

Ingredients:

- 2 large sweet potatoes
- 2 tablespoons cornstarch
- 2 tablespoons olive oil

- 1 teaspoon paprika (optional, for extra flavor)
- Salt and pepper to taste
- Optional seasoning variations: garlic powder, cayenne pepper, smoked paprika, or rosemary

Instructions:

1. **Preheat the Oven:** Preheat your oven to 425°F (220°C). Line a baking sheet with parchment paper to prevent sticking and ease cleanup.

2. **Peel and Cut the Sweet Potatoes:** Begin by peeling the sweet potatoes. You can leave some skin on for added texture if desired. Cut the sweet potatoes into uniform fries, about 1/2-inch wide. Try to make them as evenly sized as possible for even cooking.

3. **Soak the Sweet Potato Fries:** Place the cut sweet potato fries in a large bowl of cold water. Allow them to soak for 30 minutes to remove excess starch. This soaking step helps make the fries crispier.

4. **Dry and Season the Fries:** After soaking, drain the sweet potato fries and pat them dry thoroughly using paper towels or a clean kitchen towel. This step is essential to remove excess moisture, ensuring crispy fries. Place the dried fries back in the bowl, sprinkle with cornstarch, and toss until they are evenly coated. This will help create a crispy exterior.

5. **Season the Fries:** Drizzle the olive oil over the fries and season with salt, pepper, and any additional seasonings you prefer, such as paprika, garlic powder, or cayenne pepper. Toss the fries until they are well coated with the seasoning.

6. **Arrange on the Baking Sheet:** Spread the seasoned sweet potato fries in a single layer on the prepared baking sheet. Make sure there is space between the fries, so they cook evenly and become crispy.

7. **Bake and Flip:** Place the baking sheet in the preheated oven and bake for 15-20 minutes. After this initial baking time, remove the sheet from the oven and flip the fries using a spatula. Return them to the oven and bake for an additional 10-15 minutes, or until the fries are golden brown and crispy.

8. **Serve Hot:** Remove the baked sweet potato fries from the oven, let them cool for a minute, and then serve them immediately. Enjoy your crispy, homemade sweet potato frics!

Tips and Variations:

- Experiment with different seasonings and dipping sauces to customize the flavor of your sweet potato fries.
- For an extra kick, sprinkle some grated Parmesan cheese on the fries during the last few minutes of baking.
- To make sweet potato fries extra crispy, you can use a wire rack on top of the baking sheet to allow air circulation.

Crispy baked sweet potato fries are a crowd-pleasing side dish that pairs wonderfully with a variety of meals. Whether you're serving them as a healthier alternative to traditional fries or enjoying them as a tasty snack, these homemade fries are sure to satisfy your craving for both flavor and texture.

As you explore the world of appetizing appetizers, you'll find that these dishes not only whet your appetite but also serve as conversation starters and crowd-pleasers. They're versatile, allowing you to customize flavors and ingredients to suit your preferences and dietary needs. So, whether you're hosting a gathering or simply enjoying a cozy evening in, these appetizers will leave a lasting impression and set the tone for a memorable dining experience.

CHAPTER 3: Satisfying Soups and Salads

In the world of culinary satisfaction, soups and salads hold a special place. They can be comforting, refreshing, and incredibly nourishing.

Soups and salads, often celebrated as the dynamic duo of the culinary world, are more than just appetizers or sides. They are the versatile heroes of the dining table, capable of standing alone as wholesome meals or seamlessly complementing a wide array of dishes. In this section, we delve deeper into the world of satisfying soups and salads, exploring the textures, flavors, and experiences they bring to your plate.

At the heart of soups and salads lies a delicate balance. It's a fusion of ingredients that offers a harmony of contrasts: the warmth of a creamy tomato basil soup against the coolness of a crisp salad, the heartiness of quinoa and chickpeas juxtaposed with the lightness of greens, and the earthy sweetness of roasted beets harmonizing with the crunch of toasted walnuts. These dishes are a testament to the art of achieving equilibrium in taste, texture, and nutrition.

Each dish in this trio carries its unique symphony of flavors. The creamy tomato basil soup marries the tangy sweetness of tomatoes with the aromatic embrace of basil. The quinoa and chickpea salad boasts a robust blend of nutty quinoa, creamy chickpeas, and the zing of fresh lemon. Meanwhile, the roasted beet and walnut salad dances with the earthy notes of beets, the richness of goat cheese, and the toasty crunch of walnuts. Together, they epitomize the diversity of taste experiences that soups and salads offer.

Soups and salads are renowned for their nutritional prowess. They're not only delicious but also packed with vitamins, minerals, and fiber, making them a healthy choice for a satisfying meal. They're ideal for those seeking a lighter option, yet they can be substantial enough to satiate even the heartiest appetites.

These soups and salads are more than recipes; they're templates for culinary exploration. Feel free to adapt them to your preferences, dietary restrictions, or the ingredients you have on hand. Add your favorite herbs, spices, or protein sources. Swap out dairy for plant-based alternatives or adjust seasonings to suit your taste buds. The world of soups and salads is an open canvas for your culinary creativity.

Whether you're serving a comforting bowl of soup on a chilly evening, a vibrant salad to accompany a summer barbecue, or a wholesome meal that aligns with your health goals, these soups and salads have you covered. They're suitable for a casual family dinner, a weekend gathering with friends, or an elegant dinner party.

So, let the journey into the realm of satisfying soups and salads commence. These dishes are not merely sustenance; they're an invitation to savor the vibrant, nourishing, and fulfilling aspects of food. As you explore these recipes and create your own variations, prepare to discover the joy of culinary artistry, where every spoonful and forkful is a celebration of taste, texture, and satisfaction.

In this section, we'll explore three delightful options that bridge the gap between hearty

and healthy: creamy tomato basil soup,
quinoa and chickpea salad, and roasted beet
and walnut salad.

Creamy Tomato Basil Soup

Creamy tomato basil soup is a classic
comfort food that embodies warmth and
wholesomeness. This velvety soup combines
the vibrant flavors of ripe tomatoes, aromatic
basil, and a touch of cream for a silky-smooth
texture.

Ingredients:

- 8-10 ripe tomatoes (about 4 pounds),
quartered
- 1 large onion, chopped
- 4 cloves garlic, minced

- 2 tablespoons olive oil
- 1/4 cup fresh basil leaves, chopped
- 4 cups vegetable broth
- 1/2 cup heavy cream (or a dairy-free alternative like coconut cream)
- Salt and pepper to taste
- Optional garnishes: fresh basil leaves, a drizzle of olive oil, croutons, or a dollop of sour cream (for non-vegan version)

Preparation:

1. **Roast the Tomatoes:** Preheat your oven to 400°F (200°C). Place the quartered tomatoes on a baking sheet, drizzle with olive oil, and season with salt and pepper. Roast for about 30-40 minutes, or until the tomatoes are soft and slightly caramelized.

2. **Sauté the Aromatics:** While the tomatoes are roasting, heat olive oil in a large pot over medium heat. Add chopped onions and sauté

until they become translucent, about 5-7 minutes. Stir in the minced garlic and cook for an additional minute until fragrant.

3. **Combine and Simmer:** Once the tomatoes are roasted, transfer them to the pot with the sautéed onions and garlic. Add chopped basil leaves. Pour in the vegetable broth and bring the mixture to a boil. Reduce the heat to low, cover, and simmer for 20-25 minutes to allow the flavors to meld.

4. **Blend Smooth:** Using an immersion blender or working in batches with a regular blender (be cautious with hot liquids), blend the soup until smooth and velvety.

5. **Add Cream:** Return the blended soup to the pot and stir in the heavy cream (or dairy-free alternative). Simmer for an additional 5 minutes, allowing the cream to

meld with the soup. Season with salt and pepper to taste.

6. **Serve:** Ladle the creamy tomato basil soup into bowls. Garnish with fresh basil leaves, a drizzle of olive oil, croutons, or a dollop of sour cream, if desired.

Serve with: A slice of crusty bread, a grilled cheese sandwich, or a simple green salad.

Variations and Tips:

- For an extra depth of flavor, consider adding a pinch of dried oregano or a splash of balsamic vinegar during the simmering stage.
- To make it a complete meal, toss in some cooked pasta or diced cooked chicken or tofu.
- If you prefer a dairy-free version, opt for coconut cream or a non-dairy milk like almond milk for a creamy consistency.

Creamy tomato basil soup is a timeless classic that's equally fitting for cozy evenings by the fireplace as it is for casual gatherings with friends. Its simplicity is its strength, allowing the flavors of fresh ingredients to shine. Enjoy the warmth and comfort of this beloved soup on any occasion.

Quinoa and Chickpea Salad

Quinoa and chickpea salad is a vibrant and nutrient-packed dish that brings together the earthy richness of quinoa, the creaminess of chickpeas, and a medley of colorful vegetables. This salad is not only satisfying but also a wholesome choice for a light and refreshing meal.

Ingredients:

- 1 cup quinoa (uncooked)
- 1 can (15 ounces) chickpeas, drained and rinsed
- 1 cucumber, diced
- 1 cup cherry tomatoes, halved
- 1/2 red onion, finely chopped
- 1/4 cup fresh parsley or cilantro, chopped
- Juice of 1 lemon
- 3 tablespoons olive oil
- Salt and pepper to taste
- Optional additions: diced bell peppers, olives, feta cheese (for a non-vegan version), or avocado slices

Preparation:

1. **Cook the Quinoa:** Rinse the quinoa under cold water to remove any bitterness. In a saucepan, combine the rinsed quinoa with 2 cups of water. Bring to a boil, then reduce the heat, cover, and simmer for about 15-20

minutes, or until the quinoa is cooked and the water is absorbed. Fluff the quinoa with a fork and let it cool.

2. **Prepare the Chickpeas:** Drain and rinse the chickpeas thoroughly. You can pat them dry with a paper towel to remove excess moisture.

3. **Combine the Ingredients:** In a large bowl, combine the cooked quinoa, chickpeas, diced cucumber, halved cherry tomatoes, finely chopped red onion, and fresh parsley or cilantro.

4. **Dress the Salad:** In a small bowl, whisk together the lemon juice, olive oil, salt, and pepper to create the dressing. Drizzle the dressing over the salad ingredients.

5. **Toss and Chill:** Gently toss all the ingredients together until the salad is well

coated with the dressing. Taste and adjust the seasoning if needed. You can also refrigerate the salad for about 30 minutes to allow the flavors to meld.

6. **Serve:** Once ready to serve, transfer the quinoa and chickpea salad to a serving platter or individual bowls.

Serve with: Grilled chicken, tofu, or enjoy it as a standalone, light meal.

Variations and Tips:

- Customize the salad with your favorite vegetables and herbs. Diced bell peppers, kalamata olives, or avocado slices make excellent additions.
- For extra protein, consider adding diced cooked chicken, shrimp, or tofu.

- To make it a heartier dish, crumble feta cheese over the salad (for a non-vegan version).
- You can prepare the salad in advance and refrigerate it for a day. Just be sure to refresh it with a squeeze of lemon juice and a drizzle of olive oil before serving.

Quinoa and chickpea salad is a versatile and refreshing dish that's perfect for any season. Its light yet satisfying nature makes it a great option for a quick and nutritious lunch or a delightful side dish for dinner. Enjoy the fusion of flavors and textures in this wholesome salad!

Roasted Beet and Walnut Salad

Roasted beet and walnut salad is a symphony of flavors and textures, combining the earthy sweetness of roasted beets with the crunch of toasted walnuts and the creaminess of goat cheese. This salad is a visual and culinary masterpiece that's both satisfying and elegant.

Ingredients:

- 3-4 medium-sized beets (red or golden)
- 4 cups mixed greens (arugula, spinach, or your choice)
- 1/2 cup toasted walnuts
- 1/4 cup crumbled goat cheese (optional, omit for a vegan version)
- Balsamic vinaigrette dressing (store-bought or homemade)
- Salt and pepper to taste

Preparation:

1. **Roast the Beets:** Preheat your oven to 400°F (200°C). Wash and scrub the beets thoroughly. Place them on a sheet of

aluminum foil, drizzle with olive oil, and season with salt and pepper. Wrap the beets in the foil and roast them for about 45-60 minutes, or until they are tender when pierced with a fork. Once roasted, let them cool slightly, then peel and dice them.

2. **Toast the Walnuts:** In a dry skillet over medium heat, toast the walnuts for a few minutes until they become fragrant and slightly browned. Be sure to stir frequently to prevent burning. Remove them from the heat and let them cool.

3. **Prepare the Greens:** Wash and dry the mixed greens thoroughly. You can use a salad spinner or pat them dry with a clean kitchen towel.

4. **Assemble the Salad:** In a large bowl, combine the mixed greens, roasted and diced

beets, and toasted walnuts. Toss gently to mix the ingredients.

5. **Dress the Salad:** Drizzle the salad with your preferred amount of balsamic vinaigrette dressing. Toss again to ensure all the ingredients are coated with the dressing. Season with salt and pepper to taste.

6. **Garnish:** If you're using crumbled goat cheese, sprinkle it over the salad as a finishing touch.

7. **Serve:** Transfer the roasted beet and walnut salad to a serving platter or individual plates.

Serve with: Grilled salmon, roasted chicken, or enjoy it as a sophisticated standalone salad.

Variations and Tips:

- Customize the salad with additional toppings such as diced apples, pears, or dried cranberries for a touch of sweetness.
- For a vegan version, omit the goat cheese or substitute it with a dairy-free alternative.
- Drizzle a bit of honey or maple syrup over the salad for extra sweetness.
- If you prefer a lighter dressing, consider using a simple vinaigrette made with olive oil, balsamic vinegar, Dijon mustard, and a touch of honey.

Roasted beet and walnut salad is a delightful combination of flavors and textures that elevate any meal. Its elegance and simplicity make it an excellent choice for special occasions or everyday dining. Enjoy the vibrant colors and delicious tastes of this salad!

These soups and salads are versatile dishes that can be tailored to your preferences. They showcase the balance between indulgence and nourishment, offering a diverse range of flavors and textures. Whether you're seeking comfort, vitality, or an explosion of taste, these recipes are sure to satisfy your cravings and elevate your dining experience. So, embrace the world of satisfying soups and salads, where every spoonful and forkful brings delight and fulfillment to your table.

CHAPTER 4: Delicious Main Courses

Main courses are the centerpiece of any meal, where flavors, textures, and creativity come together to create a memorable dining experience.

Main courses hold a special place in the realm of gastronomy, where culinary creativity reaches its zenith. These are the star attractions of your meals, the dishes that leave a lasting impression and satisfy your appetite for both flavor and substance. In this section, we embark on a culinary journey through three delectable main courses, each with its unique blend of ingredients and cultural influences.

These main courses are more than just dishes; they're journeys through the diverse landscapes of taste. From the robust and savory Vegan Spaghetti Bolognese, reminiscent of Italian comfort food, to the zesty and vibrant Tofu Stir-Fry with Mixed Vegetables, inspired by the lively flavors of Asia, and finally to the aromatic and comforting Lentil and Vegetable Curry, a homage to the rich tapestry of Indian cuisine, these recipes promise a symphony of flavors that will transport your taste buds around the world.

Whether you follow a plant-based diet, are exploring vegan options, or simply savoring the diversity of culinary traditions, these main courses are designed to cater to a wide range of dietary preferences. They celebrate the versatility of ingredients, offering delicious alternatives for those seeking plant-powered or meatless options, as well as options for those who relish the textures and tastes of tofu, lentils, and more.In this section, we'll explore three mouthwatering main courses that cater to different tastes and dietary preferences: Vegan Spaghetti Bolognese, Tofu Stir-Fry with Mixed Vegetables, and Lentil and Vegetable Curry.

Vegan Spaghetti Bolognese

Vegan Spaghetti Bolognese is a plant-based twist on the classic Italian pasta dish. It features a rich and hearty tomato sauce with a savory blend of vegetables, lentils, and aromatic herbs.

Ingredients:

- 8 ounces of spaghetti (or your favorite pasta)
- 1 cup cooked brown or green lentils

- 1 onion, finely chopped
- 2 cloves garlic, minced
- 1 cup mushrooms, finely chopped
- 1 carrot, grated
- 1 can (14 ounces) crushed tomatoes
- 2 tablespoons tomato paste
- 1 teaspoon dried basil
- 1 teaspoon dried oregano
- Salt and pepper to taste
- Olive oil for sautéing

Preparation:

1. **Cook the Pasta:** Boil the spaghetti according to the package instructions until al dente. Drain and set aside.

2. **Prepare the Sauce:** In a large skillet, heat olive oil over medium heat. Add chopped onions and sauté until they become translucent, about 3-4 minutes. Stir in minced

garlic and cook for an additional minute until fragrant.

3. **Add Vegetables:** Add finely chopped mushrooms and grated carrot to the skillet. Sauté for about 5 minutes, allowing them to soften and release their moisture.

4. **Stir in Tomatoes:** Pour in the crushed tomatoes and tomato paste. Add dried basil and oregano. Season with salt and pepper. Simmer the sauce for about 10-15 minutes, allowing it to thicken.

5. **Incorporate Lentils:** Stir in the cooked lentils, letting them warm up in the sauce.

6. **Serve:** Serve the vegan Bolognese sauce over the cooked spaghetti. Garnish with fresh basil leaves or vegan Parmesan cheese if desired.

Enjoy with: A side salad, garlic bread, or a sprinkle of nutritional yeast for a cheesy touch.

Tofu Stir-Fry with Mixed Vegetables

Tofu Stir-Fry with Mixed Vegetables is a quick and flavorful Asian-inspired dish. It showcases crispy tofu cubes and a colorful array of vegetables coated in a savory stir-fry sauce.

Ingredients:

- 14 ounces extra-firm tofu, cubed
- 3 cups mixed vegetables (broccoli florets, bell peppers, snap peas, carrots, etc.), sliced
- 2 cloves garlic, minced
- 1 tablespoon ginger, minced

- 2 tablespoons soy sauce (or tamari for a gluten-free option)
- 1 tablespoon hoisin sauce
- 1 teaspoon sesame oil
- 1 tablespoon cornstarch (or arrowroot starch for a gluten-free option)
- 2 tablespoons vegetable oil for stir-frying
- Cooked rice or noodles for serving

Preparation:

1. **Prepare the Tofu:** Wrap the tofu in paper towels and place something heavy on top to press out excess moisture for about 15-20 minutes. Then, cube the tofu.

2. **Make the Sauce:** In a small bowl, whisk together soy sauce, hoisin sauce, sesame oil, and cornstarch. Set aside.

3. **Stir-Fry:** Heat vegetable oil in a large skillet or wok over medium-high heat. Add

the cubed tofu and stir-fry until it's golden
and crispy on all sides. Remove tofu from the
skillet and set aside.

4. **Sauté Vegetables:** In the same skillet, add
a bit more oil if needed. Add minced garlic
and ginger, sauté for a minute until fragrant.
Add the mixed vegetables and stir-fry for
about 5-7 minutes, or until they are
tender-crisp.

5. **Combine and Serve:** Return the crispy
tofu to the skillet, then pour the sauce over
the tofu and vegetables. Stir-fry for an
additional 2-3 minutes until everything is
coated in the sauce and heated through.

6. **Serve:** Serve the tofu stir-fry hot over
cooked rice or noodles.

Enjoy with: A sprinkle of sesame seeds or
chopped green onions for garnish.

Lentil and Vegetable Curry

Lentil and Vegetable Curry is a fragrant and comforting dish with the warmth of Indian spices. It features tender lentils and an assortment of vegetables in a rich, aromatic curry sauce.

Ingredients:

- 1 cup dried green or brown lentils, rinsed and drained
- 2 tablespoons vegetable oil
- 1 onion, finely chopped
- 3 cloves garlic, minced
- 1-inch piece of ginger, minced
- 1 bell pepper, diced
- 2 carrots, diced

- 1 zucchini, diced
- 2 tablespoons curry powder
- 1 can (14 ounces) diced tomatoes
- 1 can (14 ounces) coconut milk
- Salt and pepper to taste
- Fresh cilantro leaves for garnish
- Cooked rice or naan bread for serving

Preparation:

1. **Cook the Lentils:** In a saucepan, combine the lentils with enough water to cover them. Bring to a boil, then reduce heat and simmer for about 15-20 minutes, or until the lentils are tender but not mushy. Drain and set aside.

2. **Sauté Aromatics:** In a large pot or skillet, heat vegetable oil over medium heat. Add chopped onions and sauté until they turn translucent, about 3-4 minutes. Stir in minced garlic and ginger and cook for another minute.

3. **Add Vegetables:** Add diced bell pepper, carrots, and zucchini to the pot. Sauté for about 5-7 minutes, allowing the vegetables to soften.

4. **Season with Curry:** Sprinkle curry powder over the sautéed vegetables and stir to coat them evenly. Cook for a minute until the spices become fragrant.

5. **Incorporate Tomatoes and Coconut Milk:** Pour in the diced tomatoes (with their juices) and the coconut milk. Stir to combine. Season with salt and pepper to taste.

6. **Simmer:** Reduce the heat to low and simmer the curry for about 15-20 minutes, allowing the flavors to meld and the sauce to thicken.

7. **Add Lentils:** Stir in the cooked lentils and let them heat through in the curry sauce for a few minutes.

8. **Serve:** Serve the lentil and vegetable curry hot, garnished with fresh cilantro leaves. Accompany with cooked rice or naan bread.

Enjoy with: A dollop of yogurt or a squeeze of fresh lemon juice for a burst of freshness.

These delicious main courses cater to various tastes and dietary preferences, showcasing the versatility and creativity that can be achieved in the world of savory dishes. Whether you prefer a comforting Italian-inspired pasta, a vibrant Asian stir-fry, or a fragrant Indian curry, these recipes are sure to satisfy your culinary cravings.

CHAPTER 5: Mouthwatering Sides

Sides, those delightful culinary companions to your main courses, have the power to elevate your dining experience from good to extraordinary.

These mouthwatering sides are more than just accompaniments; they're a symphony of flavors and textures that elevate your dining experience. From the velvety richness of Garlic Mashed Potatoes to the crispy, caramelized charm of Roasted Brussels Sprouts and the zesty vibrancy of Cilantro Lime Rice, these dishes are the embodiment of culinary creativity.

Sides have an uncanny ability to strike a balance between simplicity and complexity. While they often rely on a handful of ingredients, it's the techniques, seasonings, and cooking methods that transform them into culinary masterpieces. From the careful roasting of Brussels sprouts to the zesty infusion of lime in rice, these dishes exemplify how simplicity, when executed with precision, can yield extraordinary results.In this section, we explore three tantalizing side dishes that promise to delight your taste buds and complement a wide range of meals: Garlic Mashed Potatoes, Roasted Brussels Sprouts, and Cilantro Lime Rice.

Garlic Mashed Potatoes

Garlic Mashed Potatoes are the epitome of comfort and indulgence. Creamy and rich, these mashed potatoes are infused with the robust flavor of roasted garlic, creating a side dish that's hard to resist.The roasted garlic infused these mashed potatoes with a depth of flavor that's irresistible. Creamy, indulgent, and deeply satisfying, they remind us of home-cooked meals and holiday gatherings.

Ingredients:

- 4-6 large russet potatoes, peeled and cut into chunks
- 4 cloves garlic, roasted and mashed
- 1/2 cup milk (dairy or non-dairy)
- 4 tablespoons butter (or vegan butter)
- Salt and pepper to taste
- Fresh chives or parsley for garnish (optional)

Preparation:

1. **Boil the Potatoes:** Place the potato chunks in a large pot, cover them with water, and add a pinch of salt. Bring to a boil, then reduce

the heat and simmer for about 15-20 minutes, or until the potatoes are fork-tender.

2. **Roast the Garlic:** While the potatoes are cooking, preheat your oven to 400°F (200°C). Cut the top off a head of garlic, drizzle it with olive oil, wrap it in foil, and roast for about 30-40 minutes until the cloves are soft and fragrant. Squeeze out the roasted garlic from the cloves and mash it into a paste.

3. **Mash the Potatoes:** Drain the cooked potatoes and return them to the pot. Mash the potatoes with a potato masher or use a ricer for an extra smooth texture.

4. **Add Garlic and Butter:** Incorporate the roasted garlic paste and butter into the mashed potatoes, mixing until the butter is melted, and the garlic is evenly distributed.

5. **Pour in Milk:** Gradually pour in the milk, a little at a time, while continuing to mash and stir until you reach your desired creamy consistency.

6. **Season:** Season with salt and pepper to taste. Garnish with fresh chives or parsley if desired.

Enjoy with: Grilled steak, roast chicken, or as a comforting side for holiday feasts.

Roasted Brussels Sprouts

Roasted Brussels Sprouts are a delightful side dish that transforms these cruciferous vegetables into crispy, caramelized bites of goodness.These petite green gems are transformed into crispy, caramelized bites of pure delight. With a drizzle of olive oil, a sprinkle of seasoning, and the alchemy of roasting, Brussels sprouts turn into an addictive side dish that balances earthy and nutty flavors with a delightful crunch.

Ingredients:

- 1 pound Brussels sprouts, trimmed and halved
- 2 tablespoons olive oil
- Salt and pepper to taste
- Optional additions: balsamic glaze, grated Parmesan cheese, toasted almonds

Preparation:

1. **Preheat the Oven:** Preheat your oven to 425°F (220°C) and line a baking sheet with parchment paper for easy cleanup.

2. **Toss with Olive Oil:** In a bowl, toss the halved Brussels sprouts with olive oil until they are evenly coated. Season with salt and pepper.

3. **Roast:** Spread the Brussels sprouts in a single layer on the prepared baking sheet. Roast in the preheated oven for about 20-25 minutes, or until they are tender on the inside and crispy and caramelized on the outside. Shake the pan or toss the Brussels sprouts halfway through the roasting time for even cooking.

4. **Optional Additions:** For extra flavor, drizzle balsamic glaze over the roasted Brussels sprouts or sprinkle them with grated Parmesan cheese and toasted almonds before serving.

Enjoy with: Grilled salmon, roast turkey, or as a satisfying side for any meal.

Cilantro Lime Rice

Cilantro Lime Rice is a lively and aromatic side dish that effortlessly elevates your meals. The fresh zest of lime and the vibrant notes of cilantro dance through each grain of fluffy rice, creating a zesty and herbaceous delight; it's a burst of citrusy freshness that complements a multitude of cuisines.

Ingredients:

- 1 cup long-grain white rice
- 2 cups water
- 1 lime, zest and juice
- 1/4 cup fresh cilantro, chopped
- Salt to taste

Preparation:

1. **Cook the Rice:** Rinse the rice thoroughly under cold water until the water runs clear.

This helps remove excess starch and prevents the rice from becoming too sticky. In a saucepan, combine the rinsed rice and 2 cups of water. Bring it to a boil over medium-high heat.

2. **Simmer:** Once the water is boiling, reduce the heat to low, cover the saucepan with a tight-fitting lid, and let it simmer for about 15-18 minutes. Check the rice occasionally to ensure it doesn't stick to the bottom of the pan.

3. **Fluff the Rice:** After the rice is cooked and the water is absorbed, remove it from the heat. Let it rest, covered, for about 5 minutes. This allows the rice to steam and become fluffy. Use a fork to fluff the rice gently.

4. **Zest and Juice the Lime:** While the rice is resting, zest the lime using a fine grater or

a zesting tool. Cut the lime in half and juice it.

5. **Add Lime Zest and Juice:** Drizzle the lime juice and sprinkle the zest over the fluffed rice. The lime zest and juice will infuse the rice with a tangy and refreshing flavor.

6. **Incorporate Cilantro:** Add the chopped cilantro to the rice and gently toss it to distribute the cilantro evenly.

7. **Season:** Season the Cilantro Lime Rice with salt to taste. Start with a small amount and adjust to your preference.

8. **Serve:** Transfer the Cilantro Lime Rice to a serving dish or individual plates.

Enjoy with: Grilled chicken, shrimp, or as a vibrant side for Mexican or Asian-inspired dishes. It also pairs beautifully with black beans, roasted vegetables, or as a base for burrito bowls.

Variations and Tips:

- For a hint of spice, add a finely chopped jalapeño pepper or a pinch of red pepper flakes to the rice.
- Replace cilantro with fresh parsley or mint for a different herbaceous twist.
- You can use brown rice or jasmine rice for a unique flavor and texture.

Cilantro Lime Rice is a versatile and refreshing side dish that brightens up any meal. Its simplicity and burst of citrusy freshness make it a favorite accompaniment to a wide range of cuisines. Enjoy the vibrant flavors and the aromatic charm of this delightful rice dish!

These side dishes are not just recipes; they're canvases for culinary creativity. Feel free to add your own twists and variations. Customize them with your favorite herbs, spices, or additional ingredients. These sides invite you to explore, experiment, and express your culinary artistry.

As you delve into the world of these mouthwatering sides, savor the textures, flavors, and experiences they bring to your table. They are a reminder that, in the world of gastronomy, even the smallest dish can leave the most lasting impression. Enjoy the culinary journey and the joy of creating delectable side dishes that elevate every meal.

CHAPTER 6: Sweet Treats

Sweet treats are the grand finale of any meal, the indulgent delights that bring comfort and joy. In this section, we dive deeper into the world of delightful desserts that tantalize your taste buds and make every meal unforgettable.

Sweet treats are the irresistible culmination of a meal, a moment of pure indulgence that brings a smile to your face and warmth to your heart.In this section, we explore three irresistible desserts that cater to your sweet tooth and showcase the wonderful world of sweets: Chocolate Avocado Mousse, Berry-Stuffed Crepes, and Vegan Chocolate Chip Cookies.

Chocolate Avocado Mousse

Chocolate Avocado Mousse is a revelation for those seeking a healthier dessert option without sacrificing indulgence. Avocado, often celebrated for its creamy texture, takes center stage in this recipe, providing the lushness and richness that any good mousse deserves. Cocoa powder and sweeteners join the avocado, resulting in a velvety chocolate delight that's both decadent and nutritious. It's a dessert that satisfies your sweet tooth while nourishing your body.

Ingredients:

- 2 ripe avocados
- 1/4 cup cocoa powder

- 1/4 cup maple syrup or honey (adjust to taste)
- 1 teaspoon vanilla extract
- A pinch of salt
- Optional toppings: fresh berries, chopped nuts, or whipped cream

Preparation:

1. **Blend Avocados:** Scoop out the flesh of the ripe avocados and place it in a food processor or blender.

2. **Add Cocoa and Sweetener:** Add the cocoa powder, maple syrup or honey, vanilla extract, and a pinch of salt to the avocados.

3. **Blend Until Smooth:** Blend all the ingredients until you achieve a silky smooth consistency. Taste and adjust the sweetness as desired by adding more sweetener if needed.

4. **Chill:** Transfer the chocolate avocado mousse to serving dishes or glasses. Cover and refrigerate for at least 30 minutes to allow it to set.

5. **Serve:** Just before serving, garnish with fresh berries, chopped nuts, or a dollop of whipped cream if desired.

Enjoy with: A cup of hot coffee or as a delightful guilt-free dessert.

Berry-Stuffed Crepes

Berry-Stuffed Crepes are a delightful fusion of delicate crepes and vibrant, juicy berries. These thin, tender pancakes are filled with a medley of fresh or cooked berries and a dusting of powdered sugar for a touch of sweetness. The simplicity of these thin pancakes belies their exquisite taste. The delicate crepes, filled with the natural sweetness and vibrant colors of berries, create a harmonious balance of textures and flavors. A sprinkling of powdered sugar adds a touch of sweetness to this dessert, making it the perfect canvas for your culinary creativity.

Ingredients:

For the Crepes:

- 1 cup all-purpose flour
- 2 large eggs
- 1 1/2 cups milk
- 2 tablespoons melted butter
- 1 tablespoon sugar
- A pinch of salt
- Butter or oil for cooking

For the Berry Filling:

- 2 cups mixed berries (strawberries, blueberries, raspberries, etc.)
- 2-3 tablespoons powdered sugar
- Optional: whipped cream or vanilla ice cream for serving

Preparation:

For the Crepes:

1. **Prepare the Batter:** In a blender, combine flour, eggs, milk, melted butter, sugar, and a pinch of salt. Blend until the batter is smooth. You can also whisk these ingredients together in a bowl.

2. **Rest the Batter:** Allow the batter to rest for about 30 minutes. This allows the flour to fully hydrate, resulting in tender crepes.

3. **Cook the Crepes:** Heat a non-stick skillet or crepe pan over medium-high heat. Add a small amount of butter or oil to coat the pan. Pour a ladleful of the batter into the pan, swirling it to create a thin, even layer.

4. **Cook:** Cook the crepe for about 2 minutes on each side, or until it's lightly golden brown. Repeat with the remaining batter, adding more butter or oil as needed. Stack the cooked crepes on a plate.

For the Berry Filling:

1. **Prepare the Berries:** Wash and chop the berries if needed. You can also use them whole, depending on your preference.

2. **Sweeten:** Sprinkle powdered sugar over the berries and gently toss to coat them.

3. **Fill the Crepes:** Lay out a crepe and place a generous spoonful of sweetened berries in the center. Fold the sides of the crepe over the berries to create a neat package.

4. **Serve:** Dust the stuffed crepes with additional powdered sugar if desired. Serve them warm.

Enjoy with: A drizzle of chocolate sauce, a scoop of vanilla ice cream, or a dollop of whipped cream for an extra treat.

Vegan Chocolate Chip Cookies

Vegan Chocolate Chip Cookies are the epitome of classic comfort. These cookies are soft, chewy, and studded with melty chocolate chips. What makes them special is that they are entirely plant-based, proving that you don't need dairy or eggs to create the perfect cookie. They're the ideal sweet treat for vegans and non-vegans alike, showcasing the versatility and deliciousness of vegan baking.

Ingredients:

- 1/2 cup coconut oil (solid state)
- 1 cup brown sugar (or coconut sugar)
- 1/4 cup unsweetened applesauce
- 1 teaspoon vanilla extract
- 2 cups all-purpose flour
- 1 teaspoon baking soda
- 1/2 teaspoon salt
- 1 cup vegan chocolate chips

Preparation:

1. **Preheat and Prepare:** Preheat your oven to 350°F (175°C) and line a baking sheet with parchment paper.

2. **Cream Wet Ingredients:** In a mixing bowl, cream together the solid coconut oil and brown sugar until well combined.

3. **Add Applesauce and Vanilla:** Stir in the unsweetened applesauce and vanilla extract until the mixture is creamy.

4. **Combine Dry Ingredients:** In a separate bowl, whisk together the flour, baking soda, and salt.

5. **Combine Wet and Dry Ingredients:** Gradually add the dry ingredients to the wet mixture and stir until a dough forms.

6. **Add Chocolate Chips:** Gently fold in the vegan chocolate chips until they are evenly distributed throughout the cookie dough.

7. **Shape and Bake:** Drop spoonfuls of cookie dough onto the prepared baking sheet, leaving enough space between each for spreading.

8. **Bake:** Bake in the preheated oven for 10-12 minutes, or until the edges are golden brown.

9. **Cool:** Allow the cookies to cool on the baking sheet for a few minutes, then transfer them to a wire rack to cool completely.

Enjoy with: A glass of almond milk or your favorite

Sweet treats aren't just about satisfying your sweet tooth; they're about creating sweet memories. The act of preparing and sharing desserts with loved ones fosters bonds and leaves a lasting impression. Whether you're whipping up Chocolate Avocado Mousse as a wholesome surprise, crafting Berry-Stuffed Crepes for a special brunch, or baking Vegan Chocolate Chip Cookies to share with friends, these sweet treats hold the potential to become cherished moments in your culinary journey.

As you delve further into the realm of sweet treats, savor the moments of joy, creativity, and togetherness they bring. Embrace the magic of desserts, and let them add a sweet note to your meals, celebrations, and life's sweetest moments.

CHAPTER 7: Beverages and Smoothies

Beverages and smoothies are the liquid refreshments that quench your thirst, invigorate your senses, and provide a burst of vitality.They offer an array of flavors, textures, and health benefits that can cater to different occasions, moods, and dietary preferences. In this section, we dive into three delightful concoctions that offer a wide spectrum of flavors and benefits: Green Detox Smoothie, Homemade Almond Milk, and Iced Hibiscus Tea.

Green Detox Smoothie

The **Green Detox Smoothie** isn't just a beverage; it's a nutrient-packed powerhouse that's ideal for those looking to kick start their day with a burst of health. It's a harmonious blend of fresh greens like spinach and kale, paired with the hydrating qualities of cucumber and the natural sweetness of green apple and banana. The addition of lemon juice provides a zesty kick, while coconut water or water keeps it refreshing and hydrating. Optional add-ins like chia seeds or protein powder allow you to tailor it to your specific dietary needs, whether you're after extra fiber or more protein.

This smoothie serves as a fantastic breakfast option or post-workout refresher. It's a great way to boost your intake of vitamins, minerals, and antioxidants while savoring a delicious, natural taste.

Ingredients:

- 1 cup spinach leaves
- 1/2 cup kale leaves, stems removed
- 1/2 cucumber, peeled and sliced
- 1 green apple, cored and sliced
- 1 banana
- 1/2 lemon, juiced
- 1 cup coconut water or water
- Optional add-ins: chia seeds, flaxseeds, or a scoop of protein powder

Preparation:
1. **Blend Greens:** Place spinach, kale, cucumber, green apple, banana, and lemon juice into a blender.

2. **Add Liquid:** Pour in the coconut water or water to facilitate blending.

3. **Optional Add-Ins:** If desired, add a tablespoon of chia seeds or flaxseeds for extra fiber and omega-3s. A scoop of protein powder can also be added for an additional protein boost.

4. **Blend Until Smooth:** Blend all the ingredients until you achieve a smooth and vibrant green concoction.

5. **Serve:** Pour the Green Detox Smoothie into a glass and enjoy immediately.

Enjoy as: A revitalizing breakfast, post-workout refresher, or anytime you need a nutrient-packed pick-me-up.

Homemade Almond Milk

Homemade Almond Milk is an example of how you can take control of your beverages by creating a fresh, dairy-free alternative at home. This almond milk recipe is not only straightforward but also allows you to enjoy the pure, nutty flavor of almonds without additives or preservatives. Soaking raw almonds overnight softens them, making them easier to blend and extract their creamy essence. The result is a silky-smooth almond milk that can rival any store-bought counterpart.

Whether you're lactose intolerant, vegan, or simply seeking a wholesome milk alternative, homemade almond milk is a versatile addition to your kitchen. It can enhance your morning coffee, create a base for nutritious smoothies, or be enjoyed as a refreshing drink on its own.

Ingredients:

- 1 cup raw almonds
- 4 cups filtered water
- Sweetener of choice (optional): 1-2 tablespoons honey, maple syrup, or a couple of pitted dates
- 1 teaspoon vanilla extract (optional)
- A pinch of salt

Preparation:

1. **Soak Almonds:** Place the raw almonds in a bowl and cover them with water. Allow them to soak overnight or for at least 8 hours.

2. **Rinse and Drain:** Drain and rinse the soaked almonds thoroughly.

3. **Blend Almonds:** Place the soaked almonds in a blender along with 4 cups of

filtered water. If you prefer a slightly sweet and flavored almond milk, add your choice of sweetener (honey, maple syrup, or pitted dates), vanilla extract, and a pinch of salt.

4. **Blend Until Smooth:** Blend the mixture for about 2 minutes, or until the almonds are finely ground, and the mixture appears creamy.

5. **Strain:** Line a fine-mesh strainer or nut milk bag over a large bowl or pitcher. Pour the blended almond mixture through the strainer or bag, squeezing or pressing to extract as much liquid as possible.

6. **Store:** Transfer the homemade almond milk to a clean, airtight container and refrigerate. It can be stored for up to 4-5 days.

Enjoy as: A creamy addition to your morning coffee, a base for smoothies, or a refreshing drink on its own.

Iced Hibiscus Tea

Iced Hibiscus Tea is a visual and gustatory delight. The deep, ruby-red hue of this infusion is only a prelude to its tangy, slightly floral flavor. Hibiscus petals, with their distinctive tartness, offer a unique twist on traditional iced tea. You can enjoy it in its pure, unsweetened form or customize it with your choice of sweetener, be it honey, agave nectar, or sugar.

This chilled beverage is a welcome companion during sweltering summer days. It provides a caffeine-free alternative to conventional iced tea, making it suitable for all age groups. The addition of ice cubes and fresh citrus slices enhances its refreshment factor, making it a go-to choice for staying cool and hydrated.

Ingredients:

- 2 cups dried hibiscus petals
- 8 cups water
- Sweetener of choice (optional): honey, agave nectar, or sugar
- Fresh citrus slices (lemon or orange) for garnish (optional)
- Ice cubes

Preparation:

1. **Boil Water:** In a large pot, bring 8 cups of water to a boil.

2. **Add Hibiscus Petals:** Remove the pot from heat and add the dried hibiscus petals.

Let them steep for about 10-15 minutes, allowing the water to absorb the vibrant color and tart flavor of the hibiscus.

3. **Sweeten:** While the tea is still warm, add your choice of sweetener (honey, agave nectar, or sugar) to taste. Stir until the sweetener is completely dissolved.

4. **Chill:** Allow the hibiscus tea to cool to room temperature, then refrigerate it until it's thoroughly chilled.

5. **Serve:** Fill glasses with ice cubes and pour the chilled hibiscus tea over the ice. Garnish with fresh citrus slices if desired.

Enjoy as: A refreshing summer beverage, a caffeine-free alternative to traditional iced tea, or a base for creative herbal tea blends.

These beverages and smoothies offer a spectrum of flavors and health benefits, from the detoxifying power of greens to the creamy indulgence of almond milk and the refreshing tang of hibiscus tea. Whether you're seeking a boost of energy, a nutritious start to your day, or a cooling sip on a hot afternoon, these drinks are your go-to options for flavor and vitality.

As you explore the world of beverages and smoothies, remember that they aren't just drinks but expressions of your culinary creativity and a means to nourish your body and soul. Whether you're embracing the detoxifying powers of greens, the creaminess of homemade almond milk, or the vibrant flavors of hibiscus tea, each sip is an opportunity to savor and celebrate the diversity of flavors and health benefits that beverages can offer.

CHAPTER 8: Plant-Based Lifestyle Tips

Living a plant-based lifestyle is not just about what you eat; it's a holistic approach to wellness and sustainability. In this section, we'll explore essential tips and insights on how to embrace and thrive in a plant-based lifestyle. We'll cover Meal Planning and Grocery Shopping, Dining Out as a Plant-Based Eater, and Sustainability and Plant-Based Living.

Meal Planning and Grocery Shopping

Meal Planning:

- *Variety is Key:* Embrace a diverse palette of plant-based foods to ensure a well-rounded diet. Explore the rich spectrum of fruits, vegetables, grains, legumes, nuts, and seeds to receive a multitude of nutrients.

- *Balanced Meals:* Strike a balance in every meal by combining plant-based protein sources like beans, lentils, tofu, or tempeh with vibrant vegetables and wholesome grains. This harmony ensures you meet your nutritional needs.

- *Batch Cooking:* Simplify your daily routine and curb food waste by adopting batch cooking practices. Prepare larger quantities of grains, beans, and vegetables that can serve as versatile building blocks for numerous meals.

- *Freeze for Later:* Harness the power of your freezer. Store excess portions of soups, stews, or cooked grains to have quick, nourishing options available during hectic days.

Grocery Shopping:
- *Read Labels:* Develop a keen eye for label reading, especially if you're avoiding animal-derived ingredients. Dive into ingredient lists to spot hidden elements such as gelatin, dairy byproducts, or animal-based colorings.

- *Shop the Perimeter: In* most supermarkets, the perimeter hosts a treasure trove of fresh, plant-based goodness. Here, you'll find your staples: colorful produce, wholesome grains, legumes, and a variety of nuts and seeds.

- *Buy in Bulk:* Consider purchasing pantry staples, such as rice, beans, and pasta, in bulk quantities. This not only cuts down on packaging waste but also delivers long-term cost savings.

- *Explore Ethnic Aisles:* Embark on culinary adventures by exploring the ethnic food sections of your supermarket. You'll unearth unique plant-based ingredients and a plethora of spices that can infuse excitement into your meals.

Dining Out as a Plant-Based Eater

- **Research Ahead:** Before stepping into a restaurant, take a moment to peruse their menu online. Many eateries now clearly mark vegan or vegetarian options, saving you time and stress.

- **Ask Questions:** Don't be shy about inquiring with your server about plant-based choices or potential substitutions. Most restaurants are accommodating and willing to modify dishes according to your preferences.

- **Ethnic Cuisine:** Broaden your culinary horizons by trying out ethnic restaurants, like Thai, Indian, or Mediterranean. These cuisines frequently offer an array of flavorful plant-based dishes.

- **BYO:** When faced with limited plant-based options, consider the "BYO" (Bring Your Own) strategy. Carry a small container of plant-based protein like tofu or tempeh to supplement salads or pasta dishes.

Sustainability and Plant-Based Living

- **Reduce Food Waste:** Make a concerted effort to minimize food waste by creatively repurposing leftovers and composting food scraps.

- **Local and Seasonal:** Give preference to locally grown and seasonal produce. This choice not only reduces the environmental impact of long-distance transportation but also supports local farmers.

- **Minimize Packaging:** Be mindful of product packaging. Opt for items with minimal packaging or those that employ eco-friendly materials.

- **Meatless Mondays:** Consider participating in "Meatless Mondays" or allocating specific days of the week for entirely plant-based meals. This simple practice can significantly decrease your carbon footprint.

A plant-based lifestyle is a powerful commitment to personal well-being, environmental sustainability, and animal welfare. These detailed insights and practical tips are your compass on this rewarding journey. They will equip you with the knowledge and confidence needed to navigate the intricacies of meal planning, grocery shopping, dining out, and aligning your choices with a more sustainable future.

Embracing a plant-based lifestyle is not only about personal health but also about making a positive impact on the environment and animal welfare. By adopting these meal planning and grocery shopping strategies, dining out with confidence, and prioritizing sustainability, you can navigate and thrive in your plant-based journey while contributing to a healthier planet.

CONCLUSION

As we conclude our exploration of plant-based lifestyle tips, it becomes evident that this way of living is not merely a dietary choice; it's a profound commitment to health, sustainability, and conscious living. Whether you are at the beginning of your plant-based journey or have been following this lifestyle for years, these insights and practical tips serve as guiding stars on your path toward a healthier, more sustainable way of life.

By carefully planning your meals and grocery shopping, you open the door to a world of flavors and nourishment. The variety of plant-based foods ensures that your palate remains delighted while your body receives a symphony of nutrients. Batch cooking and freezing offer the gift of convenience, making it easier than ever to maintain your plant-based commitment amidst life's demands.

Dining out as a plant-based eater is a delightful adventure, filled with opportunities to discover new culinary horizons. With a bit of research and a willingness to ask questions, you can enjoy delicious plant-based meals at a variety of restaurants. Even in situations where options seem limited, your resourcefulness and flexibility shine through, allowing you to enjoy satisfying meals.

Sustainability lies at the heart of the plant-based lifestyle, as it actively contributes to reducing food waste, supporting local agriculture, and minimizing packaging. The choices you make can have a meaningful impact on the environment, demonstrating that every plate of plant-based goodness is a vote for a healthier planet.

In essence, embracing a plant-based lifestyle is a multifaceted commitment to wellness and our shared planet. It's a reminder that our choices matter and that we can take conscious steps towards a healthier, more sustainable world with every meal we consume. As you embark on or continue your plant-based journey, remember that it's not just about the food on your plate; it's about the positive transformation it brings to your life and the world around you. By nurturing your well-being and treading lightly on the Earth, you're contributing to a brighter, greener, and more compassionate future for all.

In "Recipe for Plant-Based Cooking Made Easy," you'll find valuable resources and information that complement your journey into the world of plant-based cooking and living. These sections provide handy reference tools and acknowledgments that enrich your culinary experience.